Mum Alzheimer's And Me

By

Elaine Wiltshire
October 2015

With so many stories to tell over the last seven years I have always said that "I could write a book" and so I did.

This book is dedicated to my mum, who without her there would be no story to tell.

I would welcome your feedback. Please visit elainewiltshire.weebly.com if you wish to do so.

CONTENTS

EARLY YEARS

As an only child I grew up in a two bed terraced house in Kingswood, Bristol. I lived there for 22 years until I married Steve. We have now been married for 31 years and have no children.

Before I begin my mum's journey, I want to say a few things about my dad. Most children think their dad is the best and I was no different. He was very talented in many ways and especially enjoyed carpentry; in fact he built his own wardrobes and kitchen. He was also very artistic, a trait I have inherited from him as I too love to draw and paint. He was also funny, witty and had a cheeky wink (he used to wink, raise his eyebrows and grimace behind mums back) which always made me smile. I had lots of fun with him; he made everyone laugh and was always there for you. He was loved by many and I worshipped the ground he walked on. I always remember when attending school social functions being worried that my friends might laugh at dad because he had a bald head, but they never did. He was one of those people who are naturally popular and well liked.

Looking back my mum had a pretty unlucky life; she was adopted at a young age and grew up never replacing the "real" daughter her adoptive parents lost through illness. My mum married her first husband (not sure at what age), but it didn't last; mum always told me he was a womaniser and liked his drink. My mum then met my dad in Jolly's which was then based in Bristol, he was a Window Dresser and Soft Furnishings Manager, mum worked in Accounts. They married and I was born a few years later in 1962. Dad was older than mum by about 12 years, mum is 82 at the moment. I had a very happy childhood and often wish for those times back. My mum's adoptive dad died a short time after I was born but I loved visiting my little nanny; as I used to call her. My dad's mum was tall so I used to call her big nanny, she lived in a high rise flat on the third floor and I loved spending time with her or playing on the one swing that was in the grounds. It's funny but the real thing that sticks in my mind was putting the rubbish down the waste disposal shute; it's odd what you remember. My other grand-dad died before I was born. I had always longed for a brother or sister, but it wasn't to be. However next door lived a girl of similar age whose name was Karen. So began a friendship which has now lasted 53 years. In a real sense Karen is the sister I never had.

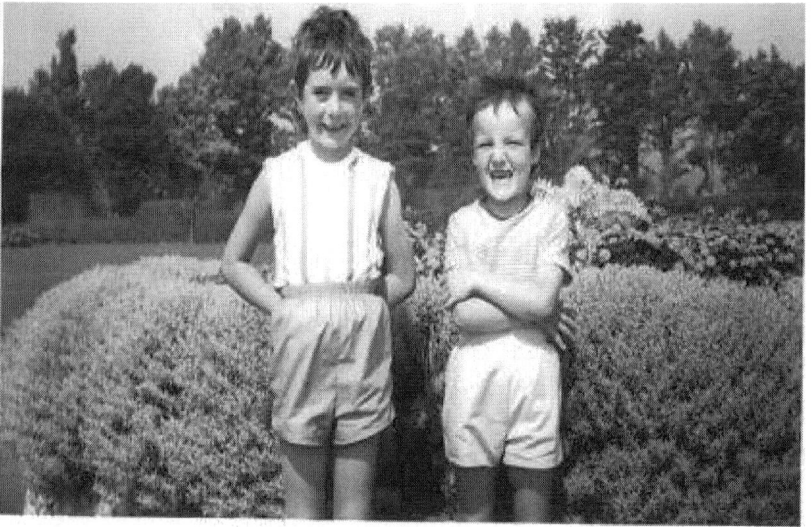

Karen (left)
Me (right)

TRACING MUM'S FAMILY

After my wedding mum and dad decided to move because it was a very "hilly" area and mum wanted to be nearer the shops and living on the flat. Mum never wanted to learn to drive and because dad was that much older she was always very conscious about how much longer dad should or would be driving. Dad didn't really want to move but mum got her own way and so they moved to a flat. A short time after this my dad had a heart attack but made a good recovery. This sudden illness came as a complete shock to us, there were no warning signs and he had always been so fit. Life in the flat continued for a few years. During this period they had a cat named Lucky – it was taken outdoors on a lead! The flat was beautifully decorated but I never felt it was the right place for mum and dad to live. Ironically the name of the cat did not affect family life, things did not seem lucky over the coming years.

My parents had a happy marriage but at the back of mum's mind she had always wondered about her birth place and her family history. I am not very good at remembering the year in which some events happened but I do remember that her opportunity came about when she had been listening to a radio programme about tracing ancestry. From recollection mum had never been in a position to be able to trace her biological parents. A change in the law made it possible to begin some research. So together we visited the central library most weekends and after months of searching we found that mums real parents had already passed away but she had two half sisters and a half brother. We managed to get in touch with two of the half sisters (the brother lived in Australia) but sadly after a few enjoyable visits things didn't work out and the reconciliation was short lived.

DAD'S DIAGNOSIS

Around 1998 my dad was sadly diagnosed with vascular dementia. Mum was his main carer and looked after him for many years. At times my life was a living hell too; the stress of it all took its toll on my poor mum who subsequently vented her feelings on me. (I use the term poor mum because now I am going through the same I know exactly what it feels like).

I had years of phone calls with mum screaming hysterically that she couldn't cope with dad anymore. I remember her arguing with him and trying to put him right all the time which always seemed to make things worse. Looking back perhaps I learned a lesson from those earlier years, I could not possibly know what was to become a reality in my life in future years. It's an interesting observation but I try never to argue with mum now. My dad was usually always very quiet and not opinionated at all. What I know is that the situation made it impossible for mum to get enough sleep. This in turn affected her ability to cope. Many times I used to go home and just cry my heart out wishing it would all just go away. Being a daddy's girl I felt I always wanted to take his side.

Living at the flat didn't last very long; it was on the ground floor and dad used to get very bad nights being restless, very unsettled and shouting etc. As a consequence another move was on the cards because mum was worried about the noise level affecting the people living above.

They decided to sell up and move to a one bed bungalow. It was a lovely little home, perfect for them with a nice little garden which they had missed (it used to be my dad's brother's property strangely enough) - my lovely Auntie Grace and Uncle Stan. My uncle had sadly passed away a few years previously and my auntie had moved out to live with her daughter as she was practically blind. As sad as this was, I felt that my dad's brother's passing had in effect "made room" for my mum and dad in their time of need.

Two single beds were bought and squeezed into their bedroom and we hoped this would give mum a better night's sleep but it didn't help at all and mum was still getting little rest. There was not a spare room and mum still struggled to manage.

LOSING DAD

Unfortunately dad only enjoyed a few years at the bungalow because in May 2004 he sadly passed away. He had gone into respite care to give mum a few days break. It was another heart attack. I can vividly remember my last time of seeing him like it was only yesterday. It was a sunny, Sunday afternoon and dad seemed absolutely fine, he was making me laugh as usual. I knew that he had eaten lunch because he still had the gravy around his mouth; he told me he had had stew. We had a lovely visit but within half an hour of me returning home we received a call to say that an ambulance had been called - he had been found collapsed in the bathroom. By the time we got there the crew were still working on him but he died a very short time after. I was heartbroken; I loved my dad so much.

I miss him still so much but have many happy memories and so many funny tales. One that always stays in my mind is when we were preparing for dad to go into respite; we had bought some name labels to sew into his clothes. Dad was trying to help out; he was sewing a label and somehow managed to cut through the trousers at the same time. He then tried to cover his mistake from mum, which left Steve and me both laughing. To this day when we see a pair of open scissors it always reminds us of my dad and "snip snip". Mum was none the wiser about what had happened; it was our secret or he would have been in trouble!

After dad passed away mum was then able to have the hip replacement she needed which was a success. We took her away on holiday a few times as she had never been able to go because she had been looking after dad. On returning home from the second holiday mum decided to get a cat – Sammie who has remained devoted to her despite how she is now. She still always follows mum into the bedroom and sleeps on her bed.

MUM'S JOURNEY BEGINS

Now I will take you back to that awful day in May 2008 when both our lives changed forever. I still remember it like it was yesterday. I had been trying to get hold of mum but she wasn't picking up the phone so I rang her neighbour and asked her to pop in to check she was alright. She found mum conscious but covered with vomit in bed. The nightmare began. I rang 999 and the paramedics were on the scene pretty swiftly, they put her on a drip, mum was able to speak and stand of sorts so they got her onto a stretcher and she was taken to Frenchay Hospital, this was about 6.00 p.m. Mum knew who I was but her speech was a bit slurred. A CT scan of her head at midnight revealed she had had a subarachnoid brain haemorrhage and it was life threatening. We were told that she could come through this with a reasonable quality of life or that she could be like a cabbage but realistically, they said her chance of survival was very slim. I felt physically sick. We stayed at the hospital all night and were able to quickly see mum when she was in recovery after the operation, her hair had been partly shaved and she was deathly white. We left the hospital about 6 00am.

Instantly, as you do, I started to read up about what had happened to her, it was very scary. I came across a subarachnoid haemorrhage chat forum "Behind the Gray" where you could share your experiences and ask for advice. It was mainly for people that had suffered a haemorrhage but also for carers as well. It was my lifeline for a long time and I still keep in touch with a few members now. Whatever time of day you could always get in touch with someone to share your concerns with. I didn't feel like I was going through this alone.

I kept a diary of every day that mum was in hospital; I visited twice a day every day. (I only missed an evening visit once).

Monday May 7th 2008
Mum had a normal day seeing a few visitors who said mum had seemed fine. When I found mum, she couldn't enlighten me with any information as to what had happened or how she felt. What turned out to be a total of forty eight days in hospital had begun.

May 8th
Mum had an operation at 2.00 a.m. to drain the fluid from her brain. We were told she had pneumonia; she was on a ventilator and heavily sedated. They took her to Intensive Care. We had to cancel our forthcoming holiday which should have been in a few weeks.

May 9th
No change; her blood pressure was causing concern and then her oxygen levels dropped so she was too poorly for another head scan

May 10th
Mum had a poor night, she was on full oxygen quota and her blood pressure was low, there was

a lot of fluid still coming from her brain. By the end of the day she was a little more stable but her kidneys were then giving cause for concern.

May 11th
I was told she had a stable night, her blood pressure was a bit of an issue and she was still critical. When I saw her, to me there was a huge improvement in that she opened her eyes and I was sure she knew me, she seemed responsive to my voice and was also taking some deep breaths. On the down side we were told her lungs and heart were both poor. Her body was very puffy all over due to all the fluids that had been pumped into her.

May 12th
A male nurse was looking after her overnight throughout her stay in intensive care. I always regretted never meeting him because his shift started at mid-night and finished at 7.30 a.m. so I only got to speak with him over the telephone. He sounded lovely and told me he had had a busy night with her. Her oxygen levels had dropped but she was on the maximum dose of oxygen already so this was concerning. She had a head scan which had shown an aneurysm that was amenable to coiling (this is a procedure which would be done through the groin to prevent blood from entering the aneurysm) but we were told that her chest must improve before this procedure could be carried out. By the end of the day mum was less sedated, nodding her head and responding to commands.

May 13th
I was very surprised to see mum had been taken off the sedation so soon after the procedure. She was trying to spell out "worried" and was nodding her head but when I visited later she was back on sedation because her oxygen levels were raised.

May 14th
Mum was heavily sedated and she went down for brain coiling of the basilar tip aneurysm; it was the longest few hours of my life. I didn't want to move from my bed, I just waited for the call which came at 6.00 p.m. to say she had got through it. I was jumping for joy. I went in to see her; she was still heavily sedated but thankfully alive.

May 15th
There was not much response at all, I was not sure she even knew I was by her bedside. It was a very disappointing visit.

May 16th
Mum was very sleepy with no recollection of the day or time. She couldn't remember the bungalow where she lived or her cat Sammie. There was talk of taking her off the ventilator. The consultants were in favour of trying but her named nurse felt it was too soon; obviously the consultant had the final say.

May 17th
Mum took a turn for the worse about six hours after being taken off the ventilator. Her blood

pressure and oxygen levels dropped and the consultants thought she may have suffered heart damage; they hoped they had got to her in time. We were told the bloods they had taken would tell us in twenty four hours. The doctor spoke with us very frankly that evening and said the odds were very much stacked against her to pull through and if she had suffered heart damage this would lessen her chance of survival.

May 18th
By some sort of miracle mum was fighting back and had totally amazed the doctors. We were told her heart had suffered a small amount of muscle damage. Before all this happened mum had a habit of turning up the corner of her right lip and this she did and gave me a wave. It was a moving moment for me, I was crying with happiness.

May 19th
Mum was still sedated slightly but she knew me. The plan was to give mum a tracheotomy which was done later that night. This procedure created an opening at the front of her neck so that a tube could be inserted into her windpipe to help her breathe.

May 20th
She had a restless night and was awake for best part of it but we were told this is quite common after a tracheotomy is fitted and would take a few days to settle. She was given some sleeping tablets to settle her down. Surprisingly, a little later she was quite alert and could now sit up.

She seemed fed up and wanting to go home. However she was very tired later and needed to be put on bellows (which push air into the lungs) to help her breath easier.

May 21st

Mum was sitting in a chair by the end of the day and could have a drink. They hoped to move her to the High dependency Ward tomorrow. She had a poor night's sleep and wanted ear plugs as the alarms were going off all night.

May 22nd

Mum was moved to HDU. I missed the nurses in Intensive Care, they were wonderful. We were told that it was still early days. She wasn't allowed a drink on this ward which seemed bizarre since prior to being moved she was allowed to drink. So mum wasn't happy about that.

May 23rd

Mum was very tired, fed up, thirsty and angry because she still wasn't allowed a drink. She didn't want visitors so I left.

Throughout her hospital stay I can only describe it as a rollercoaster, I couldn't wait to be by her bedside but then when I was, I wanted to go home. Some days I really struggled to get my head around what had happened and found it just too much for me to deal with. I felt totally drained.

May 24th
A bit brighter day today but no improvement, she was still very tired and complaining that she was feeling sick.

May 25th
She had a poor day, seemed very confused and not with it at all. By the time evening came she was vomiting. I was quite worried and spoke to the nurses so she was taken for a head scan at 11.30 p.m. followed by a chest x-ray. It was felt that her brain might be becoming dependent on the drain and that she may need a shunt as the pressure might be building up causing the vomiting.

May 26th
An anxious wait but the head scan was OK. Mum kept saying she was fed up and saying "Tomorrow will be no different". My later visit was poor; mum was very low and losing interest in everything going on around her.

May 27th
My afternoon visit wasn't too bad but not so good by the evening. The drain in her head had been clamped which they said would be monitored for forty eight hours and if she deteriorated they would re-consider a shunt. The nurses said things were still looking "precarious" due to lack of stability. She was sent down for another head scan at 8.00 p.m.

May 28th
Mum was sleepy which was concerning them this morning, but brighter later. I left her watching football.

May 29th
Mum was asleep for most of my visit during the day. During the evening she was at her lowest, no smile or any attempt to communicate, smile or wave.

May 30th
It was the best day mum had had, she was sat out in the chair. I couldn't believe the change .It was much more like the mum I knew. It was the only evening I didn't go in because I felt happier.

May 31st
How two days can be so different I will never know; today was awful. Mum had been vomiting, was sleepy and had a terrible headache (which they said may have been down to cerebral spine fluid leaking from the head drain). She didn't know I was there. I felt so helpless. I was worried it was another bleed but was reassured there would have been more symptoms if this were so. It just seemed a case of one step forward and two steps back!

June 1st
Mum had been vomiting again but her headache had improved and she had her sense of humour back.

June 2nd

She was still vomiting but there were no other changes. She had a chest x-ray. Although mum had come a long way there was still a long way to go. The oxygen was taken off and she was put on a moisture valve so the air was not so dry apparently!

June 3rd

I went to hell and back today, they couldn't wake mum this morning so down she went for another head scan. She slept all the time I was with her. The scan thankfully was reassuring; it was felt that her two hourly observations had made her so exhausted.

June 4th

Mum was sitting out in the chair again but she had a bad stomach this time, you just never knew what to expect. It seemed to be something all the time.

June 5th

The physiotherapists managed to get mum up on her feet three times albeit not that great, but she did it. It was like winning the lottery for me. I took some birthday cards in for her later to sign and she did it very well. I was a happy bunny today.

June 6th

Another brighter day, the cuff on the trachea was deflated because she was doing well (this was to evaluate her swallowing) and her hair had been washed which must have felt lovely for her.

June 7th
The headache was back and so was the vomiting and bad stomach. Mum was very irritable (can't say I blame her), even the nurse said she was grumpy.

June 8th
Mum was talking a bit of rubbish. She was moved to the General ward at 6.00 p.m. but she said she felt awful and was very confused and abrupt with me and wouldn't even kiss me goodbye.

June 9th
Mum had incontinence of faeces in the bed and was very distressed by it. She was very sleepy all day but her oxygen had been turned off during the day.

June 10th
It was a better day and she tolerated the voice valve for a few hours. A speech and language therapist came to assess her and then typically straight afterwards she was sick again – just as they were thinking of removing the tracheotomy so it was kept in.

June 11th
In the end they decided to remove the tracheotomy today so that cheered us both up. It was lovely to hear her speaking properly. It had

been very difficult to understand her. She could now have fluids and soft foods.

June 12th
Mum's birthday – she was 75. We decorated her bed up with balloons etc and took cake in for everyone. Mum had a good day but was worn out by the evening, feeling sick and fed up again. When she felt down and despondent it made me feel the same way.

June 13th
Well what a turn up for the books; mum had phoned a friend (Janet, her old next door neighbour) at 7.00 a.m. this morning so she could obviously remember her number. She was up and about using a walking frame but still struggling with food and feeling sick.

June 14th
Mum was disappointed with her attempts at walking, her leg was hurting and she was breathless, she was also very anxious "something would go wrong again".

June 15th
There was talk of plans being put into place for mum to go home, mum felt scared and worried about managing on her own.

June 16th
Mum was excited as she was told she may be able to go home in a week. A priest visited the ward which upset mum. She was walking well with a

walking frame. The doctor came on his rounds and told me that she had scared them on more than one occasion and couldn't believe how well she was doing. Well done mum.

June 17th
They had mum making a cup of tea today and doing some washing up in the rehab section.

June 18th
Mum was told she was due to go home in about six days. Occupational Therapy had been in touch and they were happy with things.

June 19th
Mum very confused today, she was rambling on about me being in a court case and another friend was serving her tea from a trolley during the night. Other than that she was well.

June 20th
Mum was champing at the bit now to come home but was very down and very anxious.

June 21st
I took mum to see the nurse who looked after her in Intensive Care who thought she looked great. My eyes were drawn to the spot where mum's bed had been and saw someone else there lying motionless fighting for his/her life. It made me feel queasy.

June 22nd
Mum ate and actually enjoyed a chicken leg for lunch; her appetite has been poor so it was lovely to see her eating something.

June 23rd
Mum feeling very apprehensive about coming home and so was I. Chocolates, and biscuits were taken in for all the nurses as a token of our appreciation for all that they had done for her.

June 24th
The day I never thought would happen, mum came home. We decorated her bungalow with Welcome Home banners. The Intermediate Care Team arrived within the hour, they couldn't get over the banners etc and said they had never seen anything done like that before which surprised me. She was my Miracle Mum and deserved it.

June 25th
The first day at home didn't go well; mum felt very low and was vomiting again. I rang the hospital and was told to ring her GP who came and thought she looked pale. She wasn't re-admitted but from here on life was to be an uphill struggle.

I can't thank Frenchay Hospital enough for the care given to mum. Everyone had been wonderful and between them all they had saved her life. We gave the Intensive Care Unit a donation. How sad this hospital has now closed.

WORDS OF HOPE

This is a poem that was in the ward mum was in, it was dated 1977 by someone whose mother was admitted into Ward One in 1996 suffering from a brain haemorrhage. It is something very close to my heart and I will always treasure this, the words are so meaningful.

Never give up Hope

The clouds grow dark, despair abounds,
You just don't know what they have found,
Expect the worst, are words you hear,
Unexpected things you fear,
Your heart feels heavy, your head is low,
What will happen you just don't know.
You trust in God to be your friend,
Because you need him to defend,
Your loved one lies there quiet and still,
No road ahead, only a hill,
A real hard climb looks like the aim,
To fix the spirit and the brain.
But time is there, to have and hold,
The unsure future will unfold,
It will take long, of that I'm sure
To take small steps, they'll find the cure.
Then slowly you will see the sun,
Of which you thought would never come,
You must be strong, don't see defeat,
Just smile at them, and feel the heat.
Then one day soon you'll take them home,
You'll have to watch them, they might roam,
But hold them tight, and love a lot,
And thank the Lord for what you've got.

HOME AT LAST

And so my miracle mum made it home despite having had everything stacked against her (albeit with a "dent" in her head) as I call it. The sickness continued most days which was worrying me. Because of this problem we took her for an endoscopy which was arranged on discharge from the hospital. It was actually on 28th July 2008, I can remember this date very well because it was the day that Weston-Super-Mare pier burnt to the ground. The result of the endoscopy did not show anything that was likely to be causing the sickness.

During the next year or so mum's next door neighbour (Jan) was a great help to me, I will never forget her kindness, bless her, she even cleaned up faeces which were **all** over the bathroom floor and when I say all over, I really mean **all** over.

For several years, Janet (yes same name) mum's ex neighbour also helped me out enormously, she always spent one day a week at mums, cleaning, ironing, cooking; in fact anything she could do to help which was much appreciated. So thank you Freda (I call her this as it's her middle name). I was really sorry these visits did not continue but thank you so much for continuing with the ironing for me. Her new nick-name is now Widow Twanky.

With the help of my two other very special friends, Karen and Cath, Steve and I are still able to have a holiday so we are very lucky in that respect, lots of others in our position can't. When we are away my two friends between them visit mum every day to sort her meals. Also thanks to Sheila, my mum-in-law who often visits her twice a day. I always feel it is a big "ask" on them all, but Steve and I both need to get away to recharge. When I'm away though, I rarely stop wondering what may be happening at home. One year mum decided to dispose of her food she didn't want by throwing it down the toilet; subsequently she made a very good job of blocking it.

Thank you also Karen for regularly giving me a night off on a Monday evening and sorting mum's tea etc and for always being on stand by when I have an evening out. It means a lot and I will be forever grateful.

During the first few years after the haemorrhage, mum was adamant that my dad was in a home in Cheltenham and she wouldn't have it any other way. How Cheltenham came into it I will never know, we have never been there or had any connections with the area but mum always used to say she had been to visit him on the bus. Now she accepts he is in heaven.

An obsession she had at this point in time was that her cat had gone blind. So we made up a letter with the veterinary logo on it saying that

Sammie was in good health and nothing was wrong with its eyes. Mum used to get herself so worked up about it. This idea seemed to work but then she would move on to some other problem.

I had this poem framed for mum, it's called Dented Halo; I love the words.

We have a dented halo,
Special Angels all are we
Bumped heads on heavens gates
Not time to go you see.
This special dented halo
Reminds us every day
To thank our lucky stars
We were not taken away
We could have been an angel
In the heavens up above
But were left with special halo's
On Earth to spread our love
Our halo's are not golden
For wings we all may lust
But instead a dented halo
Was God's choice of gift for us
So be proud to wear your halo
Our work here is not through
We have more love and joy to spread
And I'm spreading mine to you.

STRUGGLING ON

Mum subsequently managed to live pretty much independently in her bungalow for the next year or so but then I noticed small changes happening. She wasn't able to make decisions whilst shopping in the supermarkets; it was starting to take me three hours to get around. She was unable to choose a simple thing such as what cake she would like; I would lose her in the aisles and find her at the entrance to the store and she seemed disorientated with such a vacant look. The regular daily phone calls to me (always at 9.45 am) without fail suddenly stopped. She wasn't able to manage her finances which really concerned me as she had always had a very sharp brain for adding up, mum had come from an accountancy background. She couldn't work out how to do word or number puzzles any more and was starting to have trouble finding words. Alarm bells started to ring, something wasn't right here!

We visited her GP and she was referred to the Memory Clinic. This was an absolute disaster, mum refused to co-operate. I think because she just couldn't answer the questions and was so frustrated. The appointment was cut short and mum refused to engage with them again. Over time the situation just worsened and mum was relying on me more and more to help her with everyday tasks. I soon realised that the mum who loved to cook, bake cakes, read, keep everything fastidiously clean and who had always been just content pottering around in her own home was slipping away from us. It broke my heart and I found it very hard to accept. I felt very angry and used to get very annoyed with her when I visited because I would find just about everything pulled out of her cupboards and drawers to be left on the kitchen worktops or somewhere else in the bungalow. Most days there would be food, dirty and clean dishes, cups of tea, spilt sugar, several lots of cat food on plates which used to stink; everything everywhere looked a mess. I can remember shouting to mum "Whatever have you been doing?"

Looking back, I think because mum had always been so clean, tidy and everything had to be just so, her ways had had a knock on effect on me. I just felt annoyed with having to clear up the mess and muddles behind her all the time. If I find anything like this now (which is very rare since she rarely gets out of the chair), it doesn't bother me in the slightest it's not important but it seemed so at the time.

And so we muddled on, there were good days followed by bad and times when I just wished I could stay in bed and not have to face this any more. Mum's vomiting still continues to this day on and off. Most days when I am driving up to see her I wonder what will greet me; I often feel my heart sink when I pull up onto her drive and feel very apprehensive.

Steve and I found our social life was starting to dwindle which was our fault. But to be honest we never really felt much like going out. When I did I felt as though I was wearing a mask, coming across happy and smiley and giving a false image that everything was OK when in fact I felt at the end of my tether and just wanted to cry. I don't think friends really knew whether to mention mum or not. I started having to avoid making arrangements late afternoon because I had to be around to sort mum's meals out so it was difficult to go to any functions that were arranged for late afternoon/early evening. Lots of people have said to me they can't imagine what it's like, and this is so true, they can't. You have to be living in it.

In January 2010 we took mum to Bath for a visit, unfortunately whilst there she had a nasty fall on the cobbled stones. She was taken by ambulance to the Royal United Hospital and came home with nine stitches in her head – of all the places it had to be her head didn't it! I stayed with her overnight. Poor mum, she looked a sorry sight but was still smiling. Even now when I close my eyes to go to sleep, I sometimes get visions of the horrid mess she made of her eye. The rest of that year was a struggle. Mum told me that people were hacking into her phone, reporters were ringing her and she accused family and friends of stealing her money. 2011 saw pretty much of the same but with mum becoming much more of a commitment by the end of it.

MUM'S DIAGNOSIS

In 2012 I asked her GP to arrange another scan of her head because things seemed to be deteriorating again. Mum was not bothering to wash herself or her clothes; I often found her wearing stained clothing (which in no way would she change) or it was just hung up in the wardrobes dirty. She wasn't cleaning her teeth either.

She was struggling to understand instructions being given over the phone. At one stage I used to try to help her cook or warm up a meal over the phone. I would stay on the line until she managed to do it; sometimes I think it was mastered, other times I just couldn't make her understand what I was saying and it was impossible. In the end I had to accept she was no longer able to get herself a snack or a light meal. I even found cat food on a cracker biscuit one day which she had attempted to eat. She could at this stage still make a cup of tea; she can't now though some three years later.

She soon started to forget to take her tablets which I used to put up in a pivotal timed dispenser, she began leaving the fire on at times so we had to put it on a timer to stop her using it and she also left taps on (we had a flooded kitchen on one occasion) so we had to take away all the plugs. Phone calls were becoming hard work; mum had a hands free phone which she was nearly always forgetting to replace. Instead she just walked away from it and carried on talking. The phone was then left off the hook with me yelling at her on the other end asking her to either come back to the phone or replace the receiver. I had to keep ringing her neighbour to ask her to go in to put the phone back on the hook. The situation was starting to stress me out more by the day. A year or so later we changed the style of the phone to that of one where she had to replace the receiver so she couldn't walk away with it or put it down in some obscure place where often I couldn't find it.

By this time mum was starting to have a few falls and we had to cancel yet another holiday because she had one the day before we were due to go away and we were advised to stay with her for a few days. Steve had to drop our friends who we had arranged to go with at the airport and wave them off, which he found very upsetting.

Not surprisingly the result of the head scan wasn't good; it had shown a mixed picture of dementia/Alzheimer's. Although deep down, I was expecting this, I don't think anything can prepare you for actually hearing that word "Alzheimer's" given as a diagnosis. Mum showed no emotion or understanding as to what was being said; I just managed to hold back the tears and was sent home with lots of literature to read. No amount of reading can ever prepare you for what's in front of you and everyone's journey is different any way. I am glad I didn't know then what I know now.

After persevering for a few more months with things getting worse and finding myself with nowhere to turn and feeling more desperate, I reluctantly had no alternative other than to get in touch with Social Services (much against mum's will) to arrange for daily visits from a care company to help with mum's personal hygiene, breakfast and getting a snack for lunch. She was now unable to get into the bath so we had to get her legs measured (it wasn't a standard sized bath) and so we arranged for an electronic bath seat to be fitted. Steve made me laugh over this; he said it felt like he was measuring her in readiness for her coffin (you have to make light of situations and many tears over the years have turned into laughter), it's been our way of coping and kept us on the straight and narrow on more than one occasion.

Over the next six months or so mum was trialled on three different medications for Alzheimer's but she couldn't tolerate any of them due to vomiting so our lifeline was short lived. I was so disappointed for mum and me.

Mum became paranoid around this time that people were either in her loft or above her wardrobes. We even had to cancel her window cleaner and chiropodist because they were making her very agitated. There are never any explanations as to what causes these fixations. Mum used to say that she couldn't sleep as people were outside making a lot of noise (there never was) and some nights she refused to even get in her bed because somebody was already in it!

In June 2013 mum celebrated her 80th birthday, unfortunately with a tooth missing, which we couldn't get sorted in time for her photo shoot.

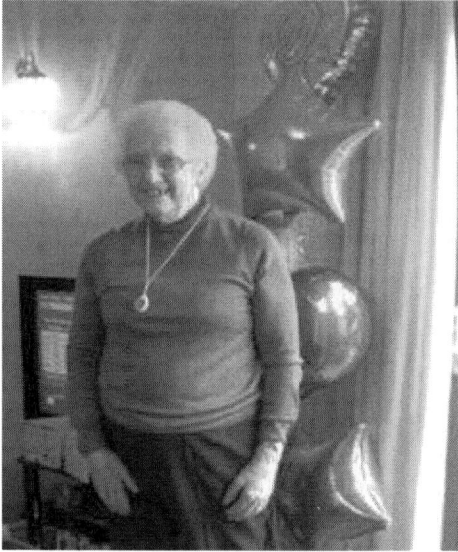

I also remember that same year taking mum out, we were walking along very slowly when we passed a lady, mum said "Would you like to adopt a daughter" I followed it up with "Would you like to adopt a mum"? The lady replied "I would rather have your mum as I don't have mine any more to look after and you should make the most of her every day!" How true these words are so to anyone reading this who are still lucky enough to have their mum or dad, just enjoy any time you can share with them as you never know when it will be your last.

In September 2013 I did the Memory Walk with some friends and work colleagues, we raised nearly £1,000. I felt proud.

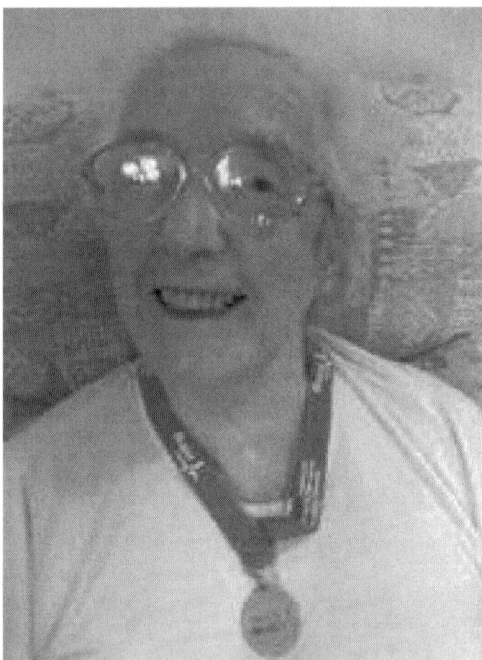

FEELINGS OF DESPAIR

During 2012/2013 I was faced with another big worry, (probably my worst yet) when mum started wandering during the night; she left her bungalow at first by her front door and just knocked on a few neighbours houses asking if she could be taken home so was safely taken back. At this point I arranged for a door sensor to be fitted which would alert me if she left the property after a certain time. Although this seemed a good idea in theory, I found myself on edge every night waiting for a call from the Emergency Call centre – relayed on to me if the sensor was activated. Consequently I was getting night after night of sleepless nights. I have been a poor sleeper for many years and this just made things ten times worse for me. I just couldn't shut off or relax.

One particular night I had a call at 4.00 a.m. saying the sensor had been activated and they couldn't get mum to answer them to confirm she was still there so I had to go up to her bungalow. I found the front door shut but no sign of her anywhere inside or out. I was frantic and immediately called the police. I can't explain how I felt, just physically sick to the pit of my stomach. After giving a brief description the police were on the case straight away, I felt helpless as they told me to stay at the property in case she returned. She didn't but then I had a call from my mum's old neighbour (Janet) from ten years ago saying she was with her. She apparently had got into a taxi on Kingswood High Street in her nightdress, coat and shoes (no money) and asked the driver to take her to her old address. Thank you driver, I never did track you down. I can't tell you how I felt when I found her; I wanted to yell and scream at her but just felt tears of relief. We de-activated the sensor; we didn't feel this was the answer to solving this problem as by the time I was able to get there, mum would be long gone.

We then decided to put up a child's stair-gate - being a bungalow and on the one level we could fix the gate across her hallway to try to deter her from going to the front door. This worked for a while but then she found she could unlock the gate to get to the front door, close the gate behind her, but then couldn't open it again to get back through so consequently she was getting stuck between the stair-gate and the front door and would sometimes be stuck there for hours. We then made the decision to get a key safe fitted outside and keep the front door locked. Peace of mind at long last.

Around this time a few of mum's friends stopped visiting; they just couldn't deal with how mum had become and found it upsetting. It's sad but just the way it is; I can understand how they felt but mum loved having visitors. It was just something else she had lost. Yes, mum had changed, a part of her brain had been damaged which controlled emotions and behaviour but it wasn't her fault. I will never judge people who have had brain injuries of any kind. Tolerance is needed on both sides.

I joined an Alzheimer's carer's group at some time during this stressful period. A small group of us have monthly meet-ups where we share our laughter, tears and other experiences. The group has been a lifeline and enabled me to meet some lovely people who are going through the same things as me. I would certainly encourage anyone needing advice or help to join a similar sort of group. I was very reluctant at first to go along and took Karen with me for moral support but I soon felt at ease and still attend to this day. I look forward to the meetings, it's where you can vent off all your feelings and share any concerns.

Mums mobility by this time had started to deteriorate; she had a shuffling gait and was very unsteady. It was time to get her a wheelchair; at first she flatly refused to sit in it but now she accepts she has to use it.

STORIES TO SHARE

There have been many stories to tell over the years, some of which have been quite funny and I would like to share some of them with you:

Mum has always been a great fan of Weston-Super-Mare, she loves the slot machines on the pier, we took her on the little train on one occasion – some of you may know the doors on the train are very narrow – well we got her in easier than we got her out I can tell you. It was one pushing and one pulling; I thought the train door was going to have to be taken off or we would be bringing her home with part of the train!

Mum's much adored cat Sammie was limping one day. Mum was whispering the word "Vet" down the phone so that the cat wouldn't hear. One of my cats had to have all of his teeth removed and mum couldn't understand why her dentist couldn't make him some teeth like she had.

This picture shows what I found in mum's garden one morning- looks like Sammie had more than her plate of cat food.

Mum wanted me to vacuum up the feathers!! Well you've got to hand it to her it would have been an easy way to clean it up.

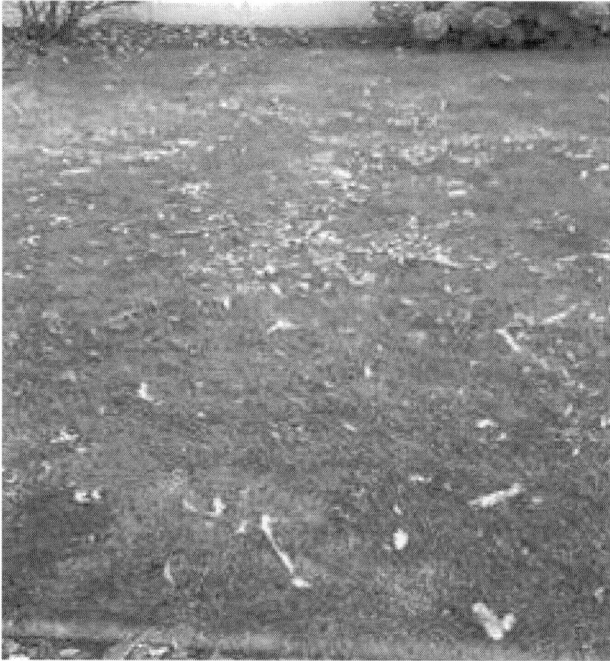

Staying on the cat theme, Sammie certainly had her five a day on this occasion. I have found all kinds of things down on the floor, but this one particularly made me laugh. I'm not sure how cats peel bananas though!

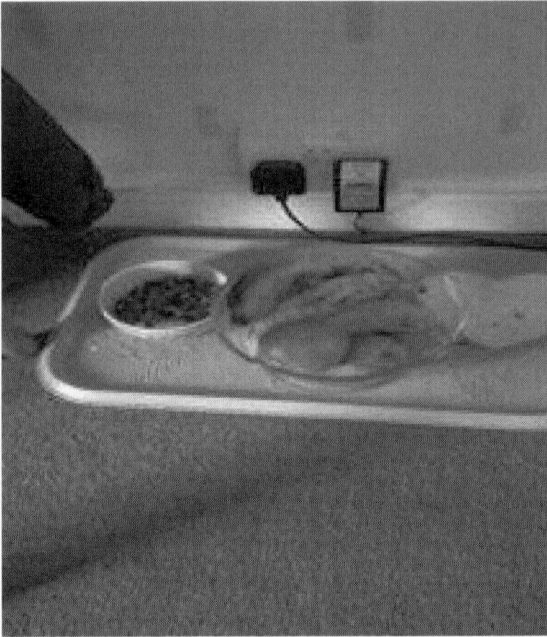

Sammie was also put on a diet and could only have an egg cup full of dried food – yes you've guessed it – one egg cup placed on the floor with her dried biscuits in, it made me smile.

We've also had Co-Co pops (cereal) in the cat's dish instead of dried biscuits. Well it is the same colour and looks very similar I suppose, very amusing. The wild birds get some odd treats as well!

Mum has a recliner chair; one evening she rang me saying she couldn't move the chair. Intrigued I had to go up to find out what the problem was. She was knitting at the time and it materialised that she had cut the remote control wire with her scissors instead of cutting the wool. We managed to get it repaired.

Mum has quite a sweet tooth, but denied all knowledge of eating a walnut whip when I couldn't get her to eat her tea. She had marshmallow all around her lips. Have a great photo of this but it doesn't look quite so funny in black and white!

I found mum in bed early one evening asking me where the vicar was to marry her and Steve (my husband).

Mum enjoys "podding" peas when she all innocently piped up with "These peas are so small, they must have just been born".

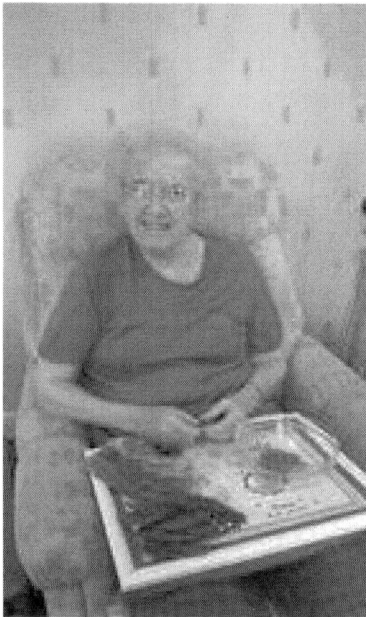

It's never unusual when mum is in a shop or restaurant to ask a stranger if they still have sex with their partner. This can be met with roars of laughter or just a stern look. It always makes me laugh anyway.

And last but not least, she enjoys throwing and catching bean bags, it really makes her chuckle. I started throwing them one day under my legs when mum said "Well at least you can still get your leg over; I can't my husband's dead".

Throughout 2014 Mum had a lot of problems with diarrhoea and sickness, it was pretty awful at times and one of the things I found the most difficult to deal with. The sickness had always been an issue ever since her brain haemorrhage and no tablet seemed to help for any great length of time; we tried a host of them. In the end bizarrely stopping the tablet she had been taking for 6 years to stop the sickness made the episodes much less frequent.

But then came the faecal incontinence, I won't go into that, it was too horrendous and I still feel traumatised by it now. It was agreed that she wasn't a candidate to tolerate any bowel prep needed for a colonoscopy or any other interventions so we had to put up with it. We had to get some incontinence pants, this was another story when one was put into the washing machine and clogged it up with the gel that they were made of, what a mess that made! I can remember on one occasion when things were pretty bad, mum asked me "Not to give up on her". All I will say is that on one occasion it looked like an elephant had been in the bathroom, I will leave the rest to your imagination! I really struggle to deal with this part of the illness.

Labelling her cupboards was the next idea though I am not sure it did any good at all (but at least the carers could find things easily). Prior to this I had been leaving notes all around the bungalow (and still do) as daily reminders; again I'm not sure any of them ever helped.

In June 2014 we think mum fell out of bed during the night, she was found by the carer the next morning with a swollen wrist and looking rather bruised. She was wearing her Piper lifeline pendent but didn't press it when she fell; yet oddly she presses it at random times asking the person on the other end to get in touch with me urgently to feed her cat or to say that she needs some help with her knitting!

Unfortunately an x-ray revealed a broken wrist so she was put into a cast (she picked blue being a Bristol Rover's fan). This was going to be six weeks of fun (not). I stayed with her for the first few evenings, and at 1.00 a.m. on the first night she burst into song singing "Oh Oh Antonio in his ice cream cart" To help things along, the carers were given more time to spend with her each morning and an evening visit was put into place.

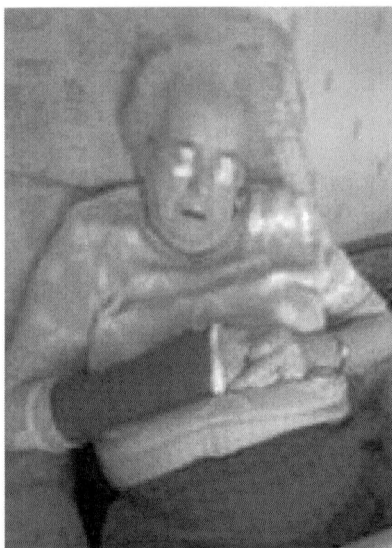

And last but not least, mum really likes Hyacinth Bucket from the sitcom "Keeping Up Appearances", it's lovely to see her chuckling away whilst watching the DVD boxed set we bought her. I have even visited a few charity shops where I purchased a few hats for Paula especially, (mum's evening carer) to wear in the hope that it might win mum around to being more co-operative and accepting eye drops/medication etc from her and make her smile — it sometimes works so Thank you Hyacinth Bucket.

I particularly love this one of mum and she looks so happy.

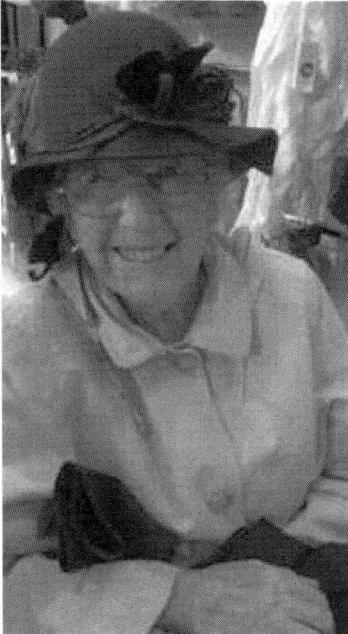

EXHAUSTION

Next came the repetitive phone calls during the day, initially it could be as many as forty in a space of three hours which was draining but to a certain extent you could ignore them. The calls each time were pretty much along the same lines, sometimes it would be to ask when I was coming up or to tell me her cat needs feeding. Other times it would be to ask what time does she go to bed and who was going to help her? Because mum kept ringing me so frequently, sometimes it took me hours just trying to get dressed in the morning. I tried ignoring them at times but it didn't stop her calling. In fact I would go so far as to say by ignoring them it made it worse. Because she used to ring me so constantly I was always on the edge of my seat and felt I should go there because she just seemed so agitated. The consequence was that I was spending five or six hours a day with her on the days I was not at work and at weekends.

But then the calls started happening during the night and I was getting night after night of disturbed sleep, I can't begin to tell you how exhausted I felt. I couldn't relax at all because I just kept lying awake waiting for the phone to ring and once she started ringing you could guarantee it would never be just the once. I was starting to get sleep deprivation and some days felt unable to function. In an attempt to resolve the problem we bought a special clock which was designed for people who were suffering from dementia. The clock gave special displays e.g. Morning, Afternoon, Evening, Night. It also gave the day of the week. However it did not prevent the calls from happening; they still continued.

My way of getting around this problem was by not having my answer phone message cutting in during the day. Instead I recorded a message tailored specifically for my mum that I switched on after 11.00 p.m. at night which would tell mum to go back to bed and that I would speak to her in the morning. I just had to remember to turn the answer phone off in the morning or anyone ringing me up during the daytime would get the message to go back to bed (which did happen sometimes and caused a few laughs).

This helped to a certain extent in as much as I didn't have to answer the phone but I could still hear it ringing so it was disturbing my sleep. Messages would be left like "You need to come up here now, the cat is very ill", often she would be quite abusive and swear saying things such as "I don't want to bloody see you ever again; you are absolutely vile and nasty". I've had messages telling me "I will never vote for you or your old man ever again" or "I will never work for you again".

I felt exhausted; it was happening most nights, sometimes only once or twice but sometimes as many as twelve and usually between 1 a.m. and 5 a.m. I had to do something and so made the very difficult decision of blocking her number between

11.00 p.m. and 6.00 a.m. – she could still ring but I couldn't hear it. BINGO – a more restful night's sleep at last without lying awake waiting for the phone to ring. Believe me you so need your sleep to deal with the day ahead so don't feel guilty about doing this if you ever have to, although I have to admit I did at first. Try to think of yourself, you need your rest. Getting sleep is very important.

CHRISTMAS DAY 2014

Christmas Day wasn't a particularly good one. I always cook the lunch at my house for both our mums. I drove to mum's to pick her up; she complained all the way down, she didn't want to come. She didn't want to get out of the car but when I eventually got her into our house she was very, very discontented and nasty. She kept shouting "Take me home, I hate it here" and she started mimicking my mother-in-law who was trying to console me as by this time I was getting upset. We pacified her by putting on some music, giving her a few presents and her mood changed. Within a few hours she was asking to go back home but at least we were able to sit around the table though my lunch went down in lumps! Never again, for any remaining years mum is with us I will cook lunch at her place. Needless to say we no longer enjoy celebrating the New Year in our traditional family fashion because we know the coming New Year will probably be very difficult to enjoy.

JANUARY 2015

At the start of January 2015 I shared a very mixed feeling moment or so with mum. She suddenly started to get very upset; wanted to hold my hand and for me to put my head in her lap (you rarely see her show any emotion these days other than anger that is). When I asked her what was wrong she said "It's because one day I will lose you", she started to smooth my hair. I tried to explain that the carers had to come in if she still wanted to carry on living at home. She told me she understood that and would always be very grateful. For a very short space of time I felt I had my mum back but minutes later it was like the conversation had never happened. I will always treasure that special moment.

The next few months saw mum getting very fixated on death, firstly it was with her cat, then it was focussed on people – it did the rounds. People that left this earth for a brief time included Steve, the carers parents, herself and then one day she started telling people that I had died. I did in fact get a text message checking I was OK. RIP Elaine (that's me) and everyone else who found their way into a coffin. Lots of people have gone to heaven over the years.

A FALL AND REHAB

In May 2015 I found mum lying flat on her back in her hallway, I opened the front door full force hitting her head and had a hard job to get through the gap; it turned out she had fallen, we think possibly after trying to pick up some post. One more job for the ever growing "To Do" list to fix a mail box on the wall outside. The ambulance crew arrived and unfortunately she had dislocated her elbow, it looked really nasty, just all withered. At first I didn't even contemplate that she had fallen purely because she spends so much time standing in the doorway. I thought she had just got fed up with waiting for someone to arrive and decided to lay on the floor in protest. Her actual body was so perfectly straight and not twisted in the slightest. I will never know to this day how she got to be in such a position.

The outcome was that she spent a few days in hospital then we managed to get her into a rehab bed in a local care home (lovely place it was too), the staff were just second to none, I couldn't speak highly enough of them. I can't say mum particularly wanted to go or settled there but we had no choice, we were due to go away within the next week for ten days so she would be in the safest place and I would have peace of mind.

And so we got to go on holiday, Hooray! I rang mum whilst I was away but most days she refused to speak to me which was upsetting but I had to dismiss it. During her stay at the home she didn't really join in much with activities and asked every day to go home. She did get up to a bit of flirting in there though with a few of the permanent residents and enjoyed the Salvation Army visit; mum loves to sing (even though her voice is appalling). If she had seemed happy and contented there I think I would possibly have come around to the idea of putting her on the waiting list with a view to a permanent placement but she wasn't so she came home on my return from holiday.

When we got her home, she couldn't remember her bungalow; she looked mesmerised when she first walked through the front door not recognising her surroundings at all. She was very disorientated and unsettled for about a week or so after which was understandable. I think deep down though she missed the company and hustle and bustle of everything going on in the home but she would never admit to this.

ODD BEHAVIOUR

You never know quite what to expect looking after someone like my mum, the days can fluctuate so much but you can guarantee there will always be something new to face around the corner. Low and behold there was, mum started to bang her bedroom window frantically shouting for help, naked. The neighbour next door didn't know where to put himself. People with dementia wouldn't think to pull down the blind or pull the curtains but it can be equally embarrassing for others as well as the person with dementia. We were looking into getting some privacy window film fitted (where mum could still see out but others can't see in) but on looking into this further, apparently when it is dark outside and the lights are on inside, people outside can still see in so we have put this idea on hold for the time being. There is no easy answer to getting around this.

Mum loves to go out, the complete opposite of how she used to be, she was always very much a home bird. Now she will wait by the front door, in her coat and shoes sometimes for hours on end; you need to go very careful when opening her front door because nine times out of ten she will be there lurking behind the door. When you take her out you can guarantee that by the time you get to the top of the road, she wants to go back home again so I never venture very far with her.

Suddenly mum got into the habit of putting items by the front the door, her explanation for doing this was that she was moving home. On several occasions I found an odd selection of items which included the cat basket, numerous pairs of shoes, knitting, cat food, purse, sandwiches, cat biscuits etc.

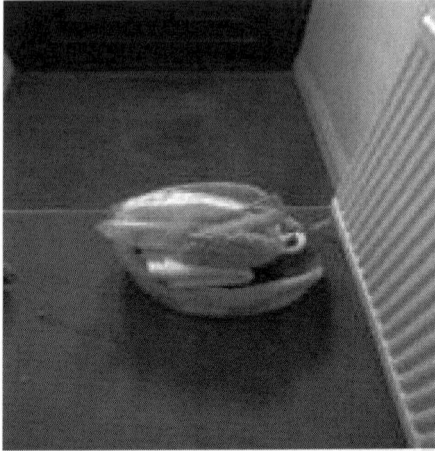

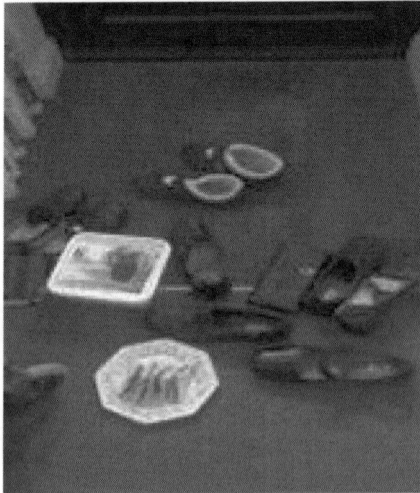

HAPPY MEMORIES

Here are a few pictures that will always make me smile.

This was taken in the care home whilst celebrating a Bristol Rover's win of which mum has always been a fan. Up the Gas Heads
.

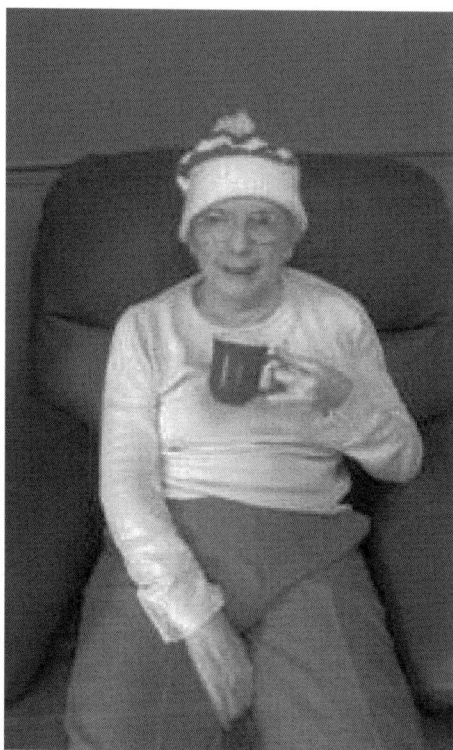

Mum had a win on the raffle at the nursing home where she went for rehabilitation after dislocating her elbow. We joined them for their open day. I had to tell her it was a scout fete to get her to agree to go.

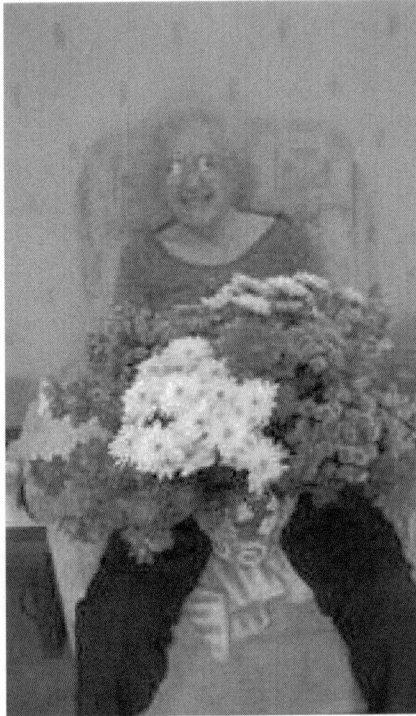

Ready, Steady Go!!!!! Mum debating whether to attempt the skateboarding park.

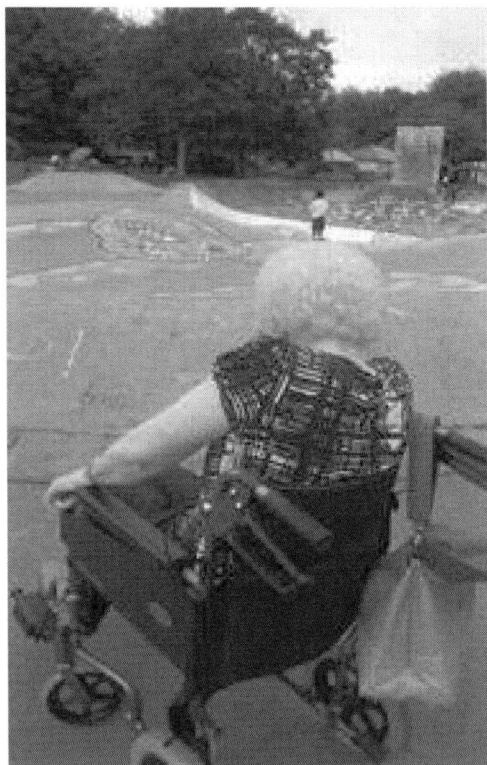

This was how I found mum behind the door one day.

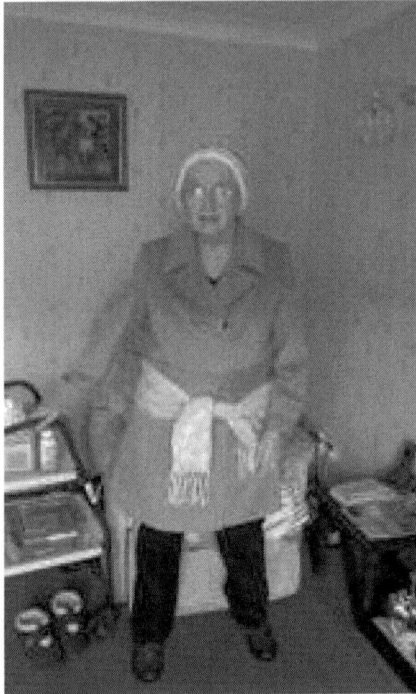

This was taken when she went through the spell of putting on her coat and shoes and just waiting by the door for someone to arrive. I invested in a wipe clean board, writing the days and times when she was going to be taken out on it but it was a complete waste of time. She still waits by the front door.

WHAT TO EXPECT

The displaying of unusual behaviour from your loved ones with Alzheimer's or dementia can be very distressing and I think I have experienced a mixed bag of just about everything. This poem just about sums it up for me.

Alzheimer's Poem

Do not ask me to remember
Do not try to make me understand.
Let me rest and know you're with me.
Kiss my cheek and hold my hand.
I'm confused beyond your concept.
I am sad and sick and lost.
All I know is that I need you to be with me at all cost.
Do not lose your patience with me.
Do not scold or curse my cry.
I can't help the way I'm acting,
Can't be different though I try.
Just remember that I need you,
That the best of me is gone.
Please don't fail to stand beside me,
Love me till my life is done.

It can also be very challenging; you will find that somehow you find the patience you could never imagine having. One of the best tips, which I have to admit I often struggled to put into practice, is to walk away from the situation when it's becoming confrontational – never argue or

61

raise your voice. It is always best to agree with whatever they are saying or try to change the subject. One way I get around this is by putting on sing along music which immediately starts her joining in and what was happening two minutes before is often totally forgotten.

I do not look forward to taking mum out sometimes because she can become very personal with strangers i.e. if I see a largely built person coming towards me I try to change my direction because mum will shout out "He/she's fat" or "My God look at the size of him/her". You can't expect people to make allowances because they don't know the circumstances but I do get very embarrassed at times and try to avoid these situations whenever possible. Mum always wants to hold my hand when sitting in the wheelchair. I think this might be because she feels safe and less anxious or maybe she just thinks she might fall out of the chair when she hits a bump! We do need our "L" plates up sometimes. She will always ask where I am if she can't see me.

When mum goes to bed each night she no longer likes the light to be turned off. Maybe it's because she feels insecure in a darkened room, there are so many situations when I wish I could understand why she feels or behaves the way she does.

Before mum had her brain haemorrhage she was never racist in the slightest but now if she sees people of ethnic origin she will talk or shout extremely loudly saying "They don't live here, why are they here?" It makes me feel very uncomfortable and again I try to avoid these situations. Unfortunately this is a behavioural trait associated with Alzheimer's. Mum will also mimic people, repeating what they are saying in a very childish voice, which I really hate.

When in her bungalow all I constantly ever hear mum saying is "This is not my home, I don't live here", but when you ask her where home is; she says she doesn't know. This is another aspect I would love to understand. She keeps saying "I don't like it here" but wherever you take her, she doesn't seem to like it anywhere!

Birthdays and Christmas's are not much fun any more, she is always very dissatisfied with any presents that are given to her, often throwing them on the floor in disgust– this is where the child like behaviour is reflected, it is just like a little tantrum. She was always so grateful and appreciative before.

Meal times can be very stressful and it is a time that I really hate; mum's favourite meal always used to be a traditional Sunday roast but ever since she had the brain haemorrhage, her taste buds altered (it's all to do with the part of the brain that was affected). Following the haemorrhage mum moved onto sweet things; cakes, chocolate, ice cream etc but seven years on I really struggle to get her to even eat that now, her diet is very limited and it does worry me. It's become all too stressful to try to get her to eat a "proper" meal. I just let her eat what she wants when she wants; it's better than not eating anything at all but in the beginning I really struggled to adopt this attitude.

From my experience I would recommend never putting more than three different foods on a plate at any one time; it causes confusion and always give small portions. I try to make it look as appetizing as possible; add a splash of colour if you can. I tend to avoid meals like casseroles which you cannot get to look particularly appealing as it just spreads all over the plate and the presentation and volume will just put mum off instantly and she will not attempt to try it. Sometimes mum will just look at the food put in front of her and say "What do I do with this" or "I'm doing this all wrong". Just give reassurance. Sometimes I have seen her use the fork but with her finger as the knife. I find she eats better if someone eats with her and she is always very conscious of who has eaten the most the quickest and likes to be eating the same as you.

The mirror in mum's bedroom has started causing her to think that someone is following her or she can't understand why the "other person" is wearing the same and doing the same as her. If she gets too agitated by this I will remove the mirror, again this is not uncommon behaviour. She often perceives her reflection as it being another person in the room.

She often starts banging the television screen when it's switched on telling whoever is on to "Shut up" or "Stop looking at me". Sometimes she will not undress in front of it saying she is being watched. If a magazine is left lying around with someone's face on it she will say "Look at that face, it's laughing at me". It's very sad to watch and equally must be very distressing for them.

Quite a problem I have experienced with mum is one of terrible agitation and restlessness every day towards late afternoon (often recognised as sun-downing). About the same time each day mum was asking to get ready for bed (usually around 4 p.m.) Every day I had to listen to the non stop repetitive conversation, practically word for word of who would undress her, what time did she go to bed and who would put her to bed? I have had to listen to her asking me the same questions relentlessly sometimes for three hours at a time which I found immensely tedious. Mum would follow me from room to room and just keep calling out my name if she couldn't see me. This type of monotonous behaviour was one that really pushed my patience to the limit. I felt like screaming and sometimes I did!

STIMULATION

Trying to get mum interested in doing anything at present is incredibly difficult. I have spent a lot of time and effort on bits and pieces trying to get her interested in doing something; e.g. fifty/hundred large piece jigsaw puzzles, colouring-in books, bingo, snakes and ladders, dominoes, snap, sewing (for aged five+), memory cards, lego, even a typewriter because mum keeps saying she wants a job! The list is endless you name it, I've bought it, but nothing has worked. Sing along music has really been the only good buy. I've even just ordered a doll as I have read that doll therapy can sometimes help loved ones to engage. We will see.

I thought it might be a good idea to get some old photographs down from the loft which I did but she says that looking at them upsets her. The only activities she sometimes enjoys joining in with are throwing bean bags, counting coins, sorting buttons and ping pong table tennis.

She has a library of large print books and although she used to have three or four books on the go at any one time and read the same page over and over again; she rarely picks up a book now, possibly because of her poor sight.

Knitting squares for cat blankets has also become a thing of the past; her squares are more like circles at times so whereas knitting and picking up a book filled her day, this is not the case now and she gets very bored so takes herself off to bed.

She has had a few voluntary workers who up until recently have regularly taken mum out, this initially worked out quite well. Now she just seems to want to go out with me all the time and has been rather rude to the lovely ladies so the visits have unfortunately tailed off. One poor lady took mum out in her two week old brand new car a few months ago and mum christened the front seat by vomiting all over it. This lady does still happily visit.

I find I have tried my utmost with trying to put things in place for mum but invariably it just seems to backfire on me! A Day Centre did not work out; we tried on numerous occasions, mum hated "Being with lots of old people who didn't know what they were doing".

As soon as I arrive at mum's bungalow she will ask "Where are you taking me today? If it's raining, I sometimes say "Nowhere because of the weather"; she then quite rightly says "Well it's not raining in the car". Can't argue with that!

THE CARERS

The visits from the carers can be very stressful for them, mum and me. As with anyone who has this disease the same faces going in are so important but it must be recognised that this is not always possible.

The carers I have met seem absolutely lovely; mum thinks the world of Debbie, her morning regular and also has a love/hate relationship on an evening with Paula but this seems to work. Paula I am sorry you have been subjected to some horrible visits so thank you for still being happy to visit her. (I think she likes you really). Remember to duck the next time a currant bun or knitting needle comes flying in your direction! Special thanks to both of you and of course to all the other carers.

Mum doesn't like uniforms, gloves and particularly new faces. Subsequently the latter causes problems when trying to administer medication, invariably with mum ordering them out of the house shouting "Get out, you don't live here".

It's equally as important for those looking after mum to feel comfortable too and at times this unfortunately hasn't been the case. Mum's behaviour has been threatening towards a few of them on more than one occasion and subsequently one or two have said they no longer wish to visit. I can understand that but it's all part and parcel of the illness.

AUGUST 2015

Mum either just doesn't want to get up on a morning, or if she does, she will very frequently go back to bed a short time after she has been washed and dressed. It's very common therefore for the lunch time carer (or if anyone else visits first) to find mum tucked back up in bed under the duvet. Sometimes she is still fully dressed, naked or back in her nightdress. Maybe she feels safe and secure here, I really don't know! When I ask her why she goes back to bed, she tells me "Well no-one is here", "I have nothing to do". "I am happy in my bed".

I am starting to feel that mum is giving up altogether now. She eats so little I wonder how she survives. The interest to do anything is completely gone. She doesn't even want to go out with the volunteers who turn up to take her out anymore, whereas she always used to look forward to these visits. She is generally very disgruntled with life and doesn't like anything.

I have no doubt that when I am not spending time with her or I am working she is either in bed or sitting in a chair staring into space. If the television is put on for her, more often than not she will turn it off. I can't be there all the time but the existence she has makes me so sad. Her ability to write is very poor now; sometimes she doesn't even know how to hold a pen. She also seems to forget how to eat some days. Her temperament can change during a split second;

from being verbally aggressive with nasty facial expressions to being cheeky and laughing.

POOR VISION

Added to mum's problems is that she is blind in one eye (and has been since she was in her forties or early fifties). She walked through a glass door thinking it was open and the next morning found she had lost her sight. At the time nothing could be done. She was referred for cataract removal on her "good" eye (I call her Nelson which she laughs at) so hopefully once this happens her quality of life will improve and she may become interested in her books and knitting again.

She passed her pre-op for this with flying colours, I was told she would need to have a general anaesthetic. A local anaesthetic couldn't be entertained due to the high chance of her moving during the operation which would obviously be too risky. I was pre-warned that the anaesthetic could possibly worsen the dementia side of things for a while or perhaps permanently I hope this is not the case. Not sure how much more I can cope with.

The operation went ahead on 24th September. Mum had the theatre staff in hysterics, she loathes beards and typically one member of staff had one; the other was of ethnic origin and another person was rather large – just the mix I needed for mum!!

As she is blind in one eye I felt really anxious for mum that when she came around she wouldn't be able to see anything and would think she had gone blind but thankfully this wasn't the case. Not surprisingly the patch they put over her eye lasted all of 10 minutes. She was lashing out at the nurses and at me when she first came back from theatre which scared me to death, I thought the side effects of the anaesthetic had done its worst already so the relief some fifteen minutes later when she calmed down was second to none.

The Consultant came to see her after the operation and mum gave him the two finger gesture telling him he had hurt her eye. The Consultant was very amused. It was decided that mum would be better off in her own surroundings so we took her home a few hours later. I thought mum would be very sleepy for the rest of the day but she wasn't, just in a lot of discomfort. It was very difficult telling someone with dementia not to rub their eye.

The following day was the best one ever; I stayed with mum for eight hours; I just didn't want the day to end. She was knitting, watching the television and even managed to get down a step on her own. She ate her food without hesitation and was so happy. She wasn't pacing and didn't seem so agitated or keep asking me if she could go to bed. Mum told me she could see! I wanted to bottle up whatever it was and hope for the same again tomorrow. When I tucked her up in bed that night she asked me "Are you going home now?" and when I said yes, she replied "Well I am already home". It was so lovely to hear her say this when for the last few years she has been saying "This is not my home, I don't live here".

Sadly the following day was the complete opposite. Mum was not interested in doing anything, her knitting and tea were thrown on the floor; she was not happy at all but at least I will always have the memory of the preceding day. A week or so on, she still didn't show any interest in picking up a book and her initial interest in knitting again didn't last either so that has been disappointing.

THE PRESENT TIME

Mum is now under the care of the Psychiatry Team at Blackberry Hill Hospital and they have been fantastic. The visits and follow up calls from the team have been very regular. Apart from the Alzheimer's Care Group that I joined I feel it's really been the only form of support I have ever received.

A new medication was tried which seemed to lift the dark cloud that was hanging over mum (I felt as though I could have done with the same medication to try at times). After a month or so the dose was increased as it was felt there was still room for improvement but this possibly caused daytime sleepiness, lack of appetite and general lack of motivation. The dosage was therefore reduced but the downside of this was that the constant phone calls during the day and evening started up again. I even had a call from her Out of Hours care company one evening saying that mum had hit one of the poor girls in the face and punched her in the chest. This sort of behaviour couldn't continue or I could have the care company refusing to continue with her care.

I made up my mind that it was either a case of accepting that mum just stays in bed for the biggest part of the day or that she is up and about but getting distressed, restless and ringing me all the time! When this happens she can pace backwards and forwards around her bungalow for hours at a time asking "To go home" and keep getting in and out of her chair. She looks so lost and vacant, it's horrible to watch. I think I would prefer her being calm and staying in bed if I'm honest but not much of a life for her with either scenario. At the end of what can sometimes be a seven hour day with mum, the constant phone calls when you get home are the last thing you want when you often have little or no patience left.

I visited mum after finishing work late one afternoon; it was a day when she would not have seen anyone since the lunch time carer had visited. I found it particularly upsetting when mum had clearly attempted to try to make a cup of tea without success. One cup just had water and sugar in it, another just something black and I have no idea what was in a third cup. It really tugs at my heart strings when I see things like this.

Another incident then closely followed involving a Support Worker (linked to the psychiatric team) who mum did not know. She visited mum at home but mum pushed her and got rather aggressive so understandably this was reported.

A few days after this I subsequently received a call from the Specialty Doctor in Psychiatry who was by now regularly involved with mums care. He was understandably concerned about this behaviour and felt that we needed to find a means of reducing her aggressiveness and agitation sooner rather than later. He wondered whether mum would consent to being admitted to hospital for an assessment. In the end we agreed that we would see how things went over the next few days and if things didn't improve her medication would be looked at again with the aim of keeping her at home. I had pinned all my hopes on that when her vision improved, it might lessen her anxiety and aggression.

A new medication was subsequently started; it's too early to know whether this will improve the situation. Things have been hit and miss at the moment. I am hoping it will help towards the aggression she shows to the carers and that I can continue to keep her at home.

I can honestly say that the last few months have really taken its toll on me. There have been days when I don't know how I have got through them. I have felt ill at times, unable to function and emotionally drained. I long for some normality (even a few hours would be nice). I cry myself to sleep on many occasions; often dreading what the next day will hold. I would like others to experience the type of days I have just to know what it's actually like; it's so hard to explain to others. You wouldn't want many like it.

SUMMARY AND ME

I asked mum one day how she felt; she told me "Not right", "I want to be a better person", "Lost", "Sad", "Fed up", "Confused" and "Lonely". I asked her if she felt happy, she said "No". She tells me "She wants to live with me because she loves me".

I've always said that mum has had three personalities during her life time. Before her haemorrhage she was very feisty and opinionated, jobs had to be done immediately, she had no patience and wouldn't wait for anything to be done, everything had to be done immediately. She was a perfectionist in every possible way which used to drive me crazy.

Initially after her head injury she became very relaxed with everyone and everything. She didn't worry about jobs being done and was always very grateful when it was. I can tell you it took some time to get used to this.

The third personality was the dementia.

Now that the dementia has progressed I have witnessed many mood changes over a very short space of time varying from being aggressive, placid, happy, grateful, ungrateful, rude and damn right miserable. This can be the usual picture for people with this disease.

So how have the past seven years made me feel? I have always been prepared to expect the unexpected; no two days are the same. My mum has become my life; everything is centered round her and everything and everyone has taken second, third or fourth place.

I never really feel like going out any more and enjoying myself, for one I haven't the energy or just can't be bothered with the effort it takes to get myself ready and motivated. I just feel so exhausted and washed out by the end of the day, having to go out is often the last thing I need. I'm not saying I don't go out, I do but I am always on edge waiting for my phone to ring, it's very difficult to relax. I find my two much loved cats are a huge boost to me and find them very therapeutic at the end of a long day.

I don't like committing to making arrangements to meet up with friends etc because on so many occasions I have had to let people down at the last minute. When we do go out, the conversation can inevitably end up talking about mum which sometimes upsets me. In fact I think 99% of my conversation with anyone these days is all about mum as she is the centre of my world and I have very little else to talk about or things going on.

Since I have been looking after mum, I have felt every emotion under the sun, hopelessness, happiness, sadness, bitterness, anger, frustration, resentment but also a great sense of achievement. I hope others going through the same will find my story uplifting and when the going gets tough, try not to give up, even though at times you will feel like it. I have been close to it several times.

Eventually I know my mum's brain will just shut down completely which will take her away from me, it's horrible to watch this disease gradually destroying a bit more of the person you love day by day. At times over the last few months I had thought that the shutting down process was starting to happen but then it picks up a little. I hope it never gets to the stage when she doesn't know me, though I did experience this very briefly once when sat next to her. She asked me "Would you ring Elaine to ask her to come up". I said "I am Elaine" and she replied "Are you; Oh yes I know that now". I have always felt I lost my mum eight years ago. I will grieve again when I lose the mum I have now.

When friends and family ask me what I would like for my birthday or Christmas, the best gift of all would be to have my mum back. I really miss the mother and daughter conversations we used to share every day, she was always so interested in how my day had gone and where I was going out.

I can't wait for a cure to be found for this cruel, disease so that carers and their loved ones do not have to go through what I have.

On the plus side of things I have found something good to come out of this illness; as a child my mum was never one for showing me much affection i.e. kisses, cuddles etc but now every day she tells me that she loves me. I will love you until the end too Mum until finally you are released from this cruel disease that has stolen your life and to a certain extent mine.

To me you will always be "My Miracle Mum" and although the last seven years or so have been very hard and challenging its seven years that I never thought I would get to share with her. From being my mum and friend she is now the child I never had. You have made me laugh mum, and made me cry; I love you so much and I hope I have done you proud. Your devoted daughter, Elaine xx

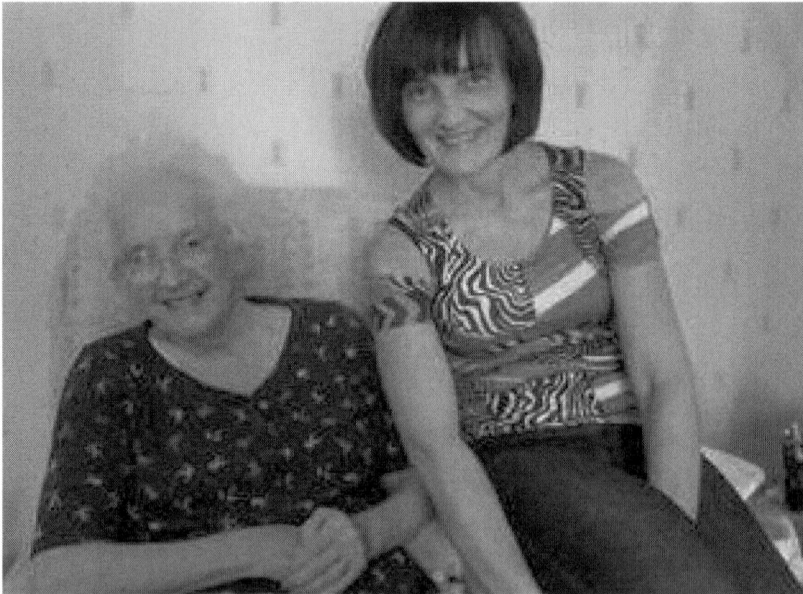

LAST WORDS

And so we will continue with life's daily challenges and struggles. Who knows what lies ahead for the months or possibly years ahead? I try not to think too much about it as it fills me with a lot of apprehension. I imagine the incontinence side of things will worsen; maybe she will not recognise others or me. Perhaps one day I will have no option other than to think about a care home (I pray it doesn't come to this). I hope the patience I thought I would never have at times and my sheer determination will be enough to keep me going until the end. I will have no regrets just a mixed bag of memories and emotions.

Finally to anyone going through the same as me at the moment or to those of you who may have to face this in the future, the advice I would like to offer is to try to keep your patience and stay calm; never argue (yes it's hard and I certainly haven't been able to put this into practice all the time). Count to ten and walk away if you need to. Music is a good form of distraction. But most importantly of all hang on to your sense of humour; it has got me through many a rough day.

If you have enjoyed my book and hopefully gained some help from it, I intend to follow it up with a second after I no longer have my mum to look after. Thank you for buying my book and sharing our journey so far and like me, try to keep smiling.